INTRODUCTION

COPD is a disease that damages your lungs over time. It may start with mild symptoms and then get worse. Treatment can help symptoms and slow disease progression. Chronic obstructive pulmonary disease, commonly referred to as COPD, is a group of progressive lung diseases. The most common of these diseases are emphysema and chronic bronchitis. Many people with COPD have both of these conditions. Emphysema slowly destroys air sacs in your lungs, which interferes with outward air flow. Bronchitis causes inflammation and narrowing of the bronchial tubes, which allows mucus to build up. It's estimated that about 30 million people in the United States have COPD. As many as half are unaware that they have it. Untreated, COPD can lead to a faster progression of disease, heart problems, and worsening respiratory infections.

What are the symptoms of COPD?

COPD makes it harder to breathe. Symptoms may be mild at first, beginning with intermittent coughing and shortness of breath. As it progresses, symptoms can become more constant to where it can become increasingly difficult to breathe.vYou may experience wheezing and tightness in the chest or have excess sputum production. Some people with COPD have acute exacerbations, which are flare-ups of severe symptoms.

Early symptoms

At first, symptoms of COPD can be quite mild. You might mistake them for a cold. Early symptoms include:

occasional shortness of breath, especially after exercise

mild but recurrent cough

needing to clear your throat often, especially first thing in the morning

You might start making subtle changes, such as avoiding stairs and skipping physical activities.

Worsening symptoms
Symptoms can get progressively worse and harder to ignore. As the lungs become more damaged, you may experience:

shortness of breath, after even mild forms of exercise like walking up a flight of stairs

wheezing, which is a type of higher-pitched noisy breathing, especially during exhalations

chest tightness

chronic cough, with or without mucus

need to clear mucus from your lungs every day

frequent colds, flu, or other respiratory infections

lack of energy

In later stages of COPD, symptoms may also include:

fatigue

swelling of the feet, ankles, or legs

weight loss

Symptoms are likely to be much worse if you currently smoke or are regularly exposed to secondhand smoke.

Emergency treatment

Immediate medical care is needed if:

you have bluish or gray fingernails or lips, as this indicates low oxygen levels in your blood

you have trouble catching your breath or can't talk

you feel confused, muddled, or faint

your heart is racing

What causes COPD?

Most people with COPD are at least 40 years old and have at least some history of smoking. The longer and more tobacco products you smoke, the greater your risk of COPD is. In addition to cigarette smoke, cigar smoke, pipe smoke, and secondhand smoke can cause COPD. Your risk of COPD is even greater if you have asthma and smoke.

Other causes

You can also develop COPD if you're exposed to chemicals and fumes in the workplace. Long-term exposure to air pollution and inhaling dust can also cause COPD. In developing countries, along with tobacco smoke, homes are often poorly ventilated, forcing families to breathe fumes from burning fuel used for cooking and heating. There may be a genetic predisposition to developing COPD. Up to an estimated 5 percentTrusted Source of people with COPD have a deficiency in a protein called alpha-1-antitrypsin. This deficiency causes the lungs to deteriorate and also can affect the liver. There may be other associated genetic factors at play as well.

Diagnosing COPD

There's no single test for COPD. Diagnosis is based on symptoms, a physical exam, and diagnostic test results. When you visit the doctor, be sure to mention all of your symptoms. Tell your doctor if:

you're a smoker or have smoked in the past

you're exposed to lung irritants on the job

you're exposed to a lot of secondhand smoke

you have a family history of COPD

you have asthma or other respiratory conditions

you take over-the-counter or prescription medications

Exam and tests

During the physical exam, your doctor will use a stethoscope to listen to your lungs as you breathe. Based on all this information, your doctor may order some of these tests to get a more complete picture:

Spirometry is a noninvasive test to assess lung function. During the test, you'll take a deep breath and then blow into a tube connected to the spirometer.

Imaging tests, like a chest X-ray or CT scan. These images can provide a detailed look at your lungs, blood vessels, and heart.

An arterial blood gas test. This involves taking a blood sample from an artery to measure your blood oxygen, carbon dioxide, and other important levels.

These tests can help determine if you have COPD or a different condition, such as asthma, a restrictive lung disease, or heart failure.

Treatment for COPD

Treatment can ease symptoms, prevent complications, and generally slow disease progression. Your healthcare team may include a lung specialist (pulmonologist) and physical and respiratory therapists.

Oxygen therapy

If your blood oxygen level is too low, you can receive supplemental oxygen through a mask or nasal cannula to help you breathe better. A portable unit can make it easier to get around.

Surgery

Surgery is reserved for severe COPD or when other treatments have failed, which is more likely when you have a form of severe emphysema. One type of surgery is called bullectomy. During this procedure, surgeons remove large, abnormal air spaces (bullae) from the lungs. Another is lung volume reduction surgery, which removes damaged upper lung tissue. Lung volume reduction surgery can be effective at improving breathing, but few patients undergo this major, somewhat risky procedure.

Lung transplantation is an option in some cases. Lung transplantation can effectively cure COPD, but has its many risks. There is a less invasive method of improving the efficiency of airflow in people with severe emphysema called endobronchial valves (EBV), which are one-way valves that divert inspired air to healthy lungs and away from non-functioning, damaged lungs. In 2018, an EBV device called the Zephyr Endobronchial ValveTrusted Source was approved by the FDA and has been shown to improve lung function, exercise capacity and quality of life for patients living with emphysema.

Lifestyle changes

Certain lifestyle changes may also help alleviate your symptoms or provide relief. If you smoke, quit. Your doctor can recommend appropriate products or support services.

Whenever possible, avoid secondhand smoke and chemical fumes.

Get the nutrition your body needs. Work with your doctor or dietician to create a healthy eating plan.

Talk to your doctor about how much exercise is safe for you.

Learn more about the different treatment options for COPD.

Medications for COPD

Medications can reduce symptoms and cut down on flare-ups. It may take some trial and error to find the medication and dosage that works best for you, but these are some of your options:

Inhaled bronchodilators

Medicines called bronchodilators help loosen tight muscles in your airways. They're typically taken through an inhaler or nebulizer. Short-acting bronchodilators last from 4 to 6 hours. You only use them when you need them. For ongoing symptoms, there are long-acting versions you can use every day. They last about 12 hours.

For people with COPD who experience shortness of breath or trouble breathing during exercise, the American Thoracic Society strongly recommends a long-acting-beta-agonist (LABA) combined with a long-acting muscarinic antagonist (LAMA). These bronchodilators work by relaxing tightened muscles in the airways, which widens your airways for better air passage. They also help your body clear mucus from the lungs. These two types of bronchodilators can be taken in combination by inhaler or with a nebulizer. Here's a list of recommended LABA/LAMA bronchodilator therapies:

aclidinium/formoterol

glycopyrrolate/formoterol

tiotropium/olodaterol

umeclidinium/vilanterol

Corticosteroids

Long-acting bronchodilators are commonly combined with inhaled glucocorticosteroids. A glucocorticosteroid can reduce inflammation in the airways and lower mucus production. The long-acting bronchodilator can relax the airway muscle to help the airways stay wider. Corticosteroids are also available in pill form.

Phosphodiesterase-4 inhibitors

This type of medication can be taken in pill form to help reduce inflammation and relax the airways. It's generally prescribed for severe COPD with chronic bronchitis.

Theophylline

This medication eases chest tightness and shortness of breath. It may also help prevent flare-ups. It's available in pill form. Theophylline is an older medication that relaxes the muscle of the airways, and it may cause side effects. It's generally not a first-line treatment for COPD therapy.

Antibiotics and antivirals

Antibiotics or antivirals may be prescribed when you develop certain respiratory infections.

Vaccines

To lower risk of other respiratory infections, ask your doctor if you should get a yearly flu shot, pneumococcal vaccine, and a tetanus booster that includes protection from pertussis (whooping cough).

DIET RECOMMENDATIONS FOR PEOPLE WITH COPD

There's no specific diet for COPD, but a healthy diet is important for maintaining overall health. The stronger you are, the more able you'll be to prevent complications and other health problems. Choose a variety of nutritious foods from these groups:

vegetables

fruits

grains

protein

dairy

Also, remember to go easy on the salt. It causes the body to retain water, which can strain breathing.

Liquids

Drink plenty of fluids. Drinking at least six to eight 8-ounce glasses of non-caffeinated liquids a day can help keep mucus thinner. This may make the mucus easier to cough out. Limit caffeinated beverages because they can interfere with medications. If you have heart problems, you may need to drink less, so talk to your doctor.

Weight management

Maintaining a healthy weight is important. It takes more energy to breathe when you have COPD, so you might need to take in more calories. But if you're overweight, your lungs and heart may have to work harder. If you're underweight or frail, even basic body maintenance can become difficult. Overall, having COPD weakens your immune system and decreases your ability to fight off infection.

Eating habits

A full stomach makes it harder for your lungs to expand, leaving you short of breath. If you find that this happens to you, try these remedies:

Clear your airways about an hour before a meal.

Take smaller bites of food that you chew slowly before swallowing.

Swap three meals a day for five or six smaller meals.

Save fluids until the end so you feel less full during the meal.

Check out these 5 diet tips for people with COPD.

Living with COPD

COPD requires lifelong disease management. That means following the advice of your healthcare team and maintaining healthy lifestyle habits. Since your lungs are weakened, you'll want to avoid anything that might overtax them or cause a flare-up. Here's a list of things to consider as you adjust your lifestyle.

Avoid smoking. If you're having trouble quitting, talk to your doctor about smoking cessation programs. Try to avoid secondhand smoke, chemical fumes, air pollution, and dust.

Work out. A little exercise each day can help you stay strong. Talk to your doctor about how much exercise is good for you.

Eat a diet of nutritious foods. Avoid highly processed foods that are loaded with calories and salt, but lack nutrients.

Treating other conditions. If you have other chronic diseases along with COPD, it's important to manage those as well, particularly diabetes mellitus and heart disease.

Clean house. Clear the clutter and streamline your home so that it takes less energy to clean and do other household tasks. If you have advanced COPD, get help with daily chores.

Be prepared for flare-ups. Carry your emergency contact information with you and post it on your refrigerator. Include information about what medications you take, as well as the doses. Program emergency numbers into your phone.

Find support. It can be a relief to talk to others who understand. Consider joining a support group. The COPD Foundation provides a comprehensive list of organizations and resources for people living with COPD.

What are the stages of COPD?

One measure of COPD is achieved by spirometry grading. There are different grading systems, and one grading system is part of the GOLD classification. The GOLD classification is used for determining COPD severity and helping to form a prognosis and treatment plan. There are four GOLD grades based on spirometry testing:

grade 1: mild

grade 2: moderate

grade 3: severe

grade 4: very severe

This is based on the spirometry test result of your FEV1. This is the amount of air you can breathe out of the lungs in the first second of a forced expiration. The severity increases as your FEV1 decreases.

The GOLD classification also takes into account your individual symptoms and history of acute exacerbations. Based on this information, your doctor can assign a letter group to you to help define your COPD grade. As the disease progresses, you're more susceptible to complications, such as:

respiratory infections, including common colds, flu, and pneumonia

heart problems

high blood pressure in lung arteries (pulmonary hypertension)

lung cancer

depression and anxiety

Is there a connection between COPD and lung cancer?

COPD and lung cancer are major health problems worldwide. These two diseases are linked in a number of ways. COPD and lung cancer have several common risk factors. Smoking is the number one risk factor for both diseases. Both are more likely if you breathe secondhand smoke, or are exposed to chemicals or other fumes in the workplace. There may be a genetic predisposition to developing both diseases. Also, the risk of developing either COPD or lung cancer increases with age. It was estimated in 2009 that between 40 and 70 percentTrusted Source of people with lung cancer also have COPD. This same 2009 studyTrusted Source concluded that COPD is a risk factor for lung cancer.

COPD statistics

Worldwide, it's estimated that about 65 millionTrusted Source people have moderate to severe COPD. About 16 millionTrusted Source adults in the United States have a diagnosis of COPD. Most people with COPD are 40 years of age or older. The majority of people with COPD are smokers or former smokers. Smoking is the most important risk factor that can be changed. In up to 5 percentTrusted Source of people with COPD, the cause is a genetic disorder involving a deficiency of a protein called alpha-1-antitrypsin.

COPD is a leading cause of hospitalizations in industrialized countries. In the United States, COPD is responsible for a large amount of emergency department visits and hospital admissions. In the year 2000, it was noted that there were over 700,000 hospital admissions and approximately 1.5 millionTrusted Source emergency department visits. COPD is the third leading cause of death in the United States. More women than men die from COPD each year. It's projected that the number of patients diagnosed with COPD will increase by more than 150 percent from 2010 to 2030. Much of that can be attributed to an aging population.

What's the outlook for people with COPD?
COPD generally reduces life expectancy, though the outlook varies considerably from person to person. People with COPD who never smoked may have a modest reduction in life expectancyTrusted Source, while former and current smokers are likely to have a larger reduction.

COPD tends to progress slowly. You may not even know you have it during the early stages. Once you have a diagnosis, you'll need to start seeing your doctor on a regular basis. You'll also have to take steps to manage your condition and make the appropriate changes to your daily life. Early symptoms can usually be managed, and certain lifestyle choices can help you maintain a good quality of life for some time. As the disease progresses, symptoms can become increasingly limiting.

People with severe stages of COPD may not be able to care for themselves without assistance. They're at increased risk of developing respiratory infections, heart problems, and lung cancer. They may also be at risk of depression and anxiety. Besides smoking, your outlook depends on how well you respond to treatment and whether you can avoid serious complications. Your doctor is in the best position to evaluate your overall health and give you an idea about what to expect.

COPD NUTRITION GUIDE: 5 DIET TIPS FOR PEOPLE WITH CHRONIC OBSTRUCTIVE PULMONARY DISEASE

A healthy diet cannot cure chronic obstructive pulmonary disease (COPD) but can help your body manage infections, including chest infections that may lead to hospitalization. Eating healthfully can make you feel better, too. Maintaining your nutrition while managing this condition doesn't have to be boring or difficult. Just follow these healthy tips.

What to eat

A reduced carbohydrate diet results in lower carbon dioxide production. This may help people with COPD better manage their health. Diets rich in whole foods, vegetables, and healthy fats, such as the Mediterranean diet, can preserve lung functionTrusted Source in COPD and even reduce the risk of it developing.

Protein-rich foods

High quality protein sources include:

plant-based sources like tofu, tempeh, and seitan

beans, pulses, including chickpeas and edamame

lean poultry

eggs

lean red meat

oily fish like salmon, mackerel, and sardines

Complex carbohydrates

If you include carbohydrates in your diet, opt for complex carbohydrates. These foods are high in fiber, which helps improve the function of the digestive system and blood sugar management. Foods to incorporate into your diet include:

peas

bran

potatoes with skin

lentils

quinoa

beans

oats

barley

Potassium-rich foods

Potassium is vital to lung function, so a potassium deficiency can cause breathing issues. Try to eat foods containing high levels of potassium, such as:

avocados

dark leafy greens

tomatoes

asparagus

beets

potatoes

bananas

oranges

Potassium-rich foods can be beneficial if your dietitian or doctor has prescribed a diuretic medication.

Healthy fats

When choosing to eat a higher fat diet, instead of selecting fried foods, opt for snacks and meals containing fats like:

avocados

nuts

seeds

coconut and coconut oil

olives and olive oil

fatty fish

cheese

What to limit

Certain foods can cause problems, such as gas and bloating, or have little to no nutritional value. Foods to avoid or minimize include:

Salt: Too much sodium or salt in your diet causes water retention, which may affect your breathing ability.

Certain fruits: Apples, stone fruits, such as apricots and peaches, and melons may cause bloating and gas in some people due to fermentable carbohydrates. This may lead to breathing problems in people with COPD.

Some vegetables: Many vegetables and legumes cause bloating and gas, including:

beans

Brussels sprouts

cabbage

cauliflower

corn

onions

peas

Dairy: Some dairy products, such as milk and cheese, make phlegm thicker.

Fried foods: Fried, deep fried, or greasy foods can cause gas and indigestion. Heavily spiced foods may also cause discomfort and may affect your breathing.

Hydration

People with COPD should try to drink plenty of fluids throughout the day. Around six to eight 8-ounce glasses of noncaffeinated beverages are recommended per day. Adequate hydration keeps mucus thin and makes it easier to cough up.

Watch your weight

Your weight can affect COPD symptoms and management.

If you're overweight

Having overweight or obesity can exacerbate COPD symptoms. Excess body weight often means your heart and lungs must work harder, making breathing more difficult. This may also increase the demand for oxygen. Your weight will affect the number of calories your body requires to function. Your doctor or dietitian can advise you on managing your weight by following a customized eating plan and an achievable exercise program.

If you're underweight

Some symptoms of COPD, such as lack of appetite, depression, or feeling unwell, can cause you to eat less and ultimately lose weight. If you're underweight, you may feel tired or be more prone to infections. People with COPD typically require more energy for breathing and other muscle functions. As a result, adequate energy intake is essential. If you're underweight, try to include healthy, high calorie snacks in your diet.

Be prepared for mealtime

With COPD, making food preparation a straightforward and stress-free process is important. Make mealtime easier, encourage your appetite if you're underweight, and stick to a healthy eating program by following these guidelines:

Eat small meals

Try eating five to six small meals daily rather than three large ones. Eating smaller meals may help you avoid filling up your stomach too much and give your lungs enough room to expand, making breathing easier.

Eat your main meal early

Try to eat your main meal early in the day. This will boost your energy levels for the whole day.

Choose quick and easy foods

Choose foods that are quick and easy to prepare. This will help you avoid wasting energy. Sit down when preparing meals so you aren't too tired to eat and ask family and friends to assist you with meal preparation if necessary. You may also be eligible for a meal home delivery service.

Get comfortable

Sit comfortably in a high-backed chair when eating to avoid putting too much pressure on your lungs.

Make enough for leftovers

When making a meal, make a bigger portion to refrigerate or freeze some for later and have nutritious meals available when you feel too tired to cook.

It's important to stay mindful of your overall health when you have COPD, and nutrition is a big part of that. Planning healthy meals and snacks while emphasizing higher fat intake can help you manage symptoms and minimize complications.

COPD and Cough: How They're Related and What You Should Know

If you have COPD, coughing is often necessary to clear mucus from your airways. allowing you to breathe more easily. Doctors may recommend a specific technique. Coughing may seem like a symptom you want to relieve, but, in the case of COPD, it serves a function.

What are the symptoms of chronic obstructive pulmonary disease?

If you have chronic obstructive pulmonary disease (COPD), you'll likely experience one or more of the following four symptoms:

shortness of breath, especially with activity

wheezing, or producing a gasping, whistling sound when you try to breathe

feeling tight or constricted in your chest area

coughing that produces moderate to large amounts of mucus or sputum

People tend to find coughing the most disruptive of these symptoms.

Coughing can interfere with social events, such as going to the movies, and prevent you from falling asleep at night. Many people go to their doctor or an urgent care center seeking relief from the chronic coughing associated with COPD.

When should you see a pulmonologist?

If you have a cough that lasts more than 3 weeks or becomes severe, your doctor may refer you to a pulmonologist. A pulmonologist is a doctor who specializes in diagnosing and treating conditions of the respiratory system, such as COPD, asthma, and lung cancer.

How are COPD and cough related?

As annoying as this coughing may be, it actually serves a useful function. Deep coughing clears the mucus that clogs your airways, allowing you to breathe more easily. Some doctors teach their patients how to cough and encourage them to do so often. Other experts even go a step further and advise against doing anything to stop the coughing, as a clear airway means easier breathing in the long run.

What causes coughing with COPD?
If you've had COPD for a while, you probably know how much you usually cough. If you find yourself coughing more than usual or coughing up sputum that looks different than it normally does, it may be time to go to the doctor to make sure you're not having a flare-up or an exacerbation. An increase in coughing can have several causes. Your body may be producing more sputum or mucus. Exposure to irritants, especially cigarette smoke or harsh fumes, can also increase coughing. You may also be coughing more because you've developed a comorbidity, which means another illness exists alongside your COPD. Examples of comorbidities include infections such as pneumonia or influenza, or issues such as gastroesophageal reflux disease (GERD). When you lie down, GERD can push stomach acid into your throat and mouth and cause you to cough.

If your increased coughing is due to a comorbidity, you may speak with a doctor about taking medications to return to your regular level of coughing. Don't make any assumptions, though — speak with your doctor as they can make a diagnosis and prescribe you the right medication.

What are the treatments for coughing?

If you smoke, the most important step is to stop smoking. Quitting will end "smoker's cough," the dry, hacking cough common among people who smoke tobacco. A deep, productive cough that clears the airways of mucus may replace this dry cough.

Drugs for coughing

Short- or long-acting inhaled beta-agonists such as albuterol or salmeterol (Serevent) will sometimes help decrease coughing. Beta-agonists are a type of bronchodilator that helps open your airways and get more oxygen into your lungs. Long-acting bronchodilators are sometimes used in combination with an inhaled corticosteroid. Advair and Symbicort are examples of combination medications. Some older researchTrusted Source has studied the effectiveness of cough syrup with codeine.

Although a few small studies showed a significant reduction in coughing, other studies could not reproduce that result. Long-term use of codeine can have potential for dependence. Using cough syrup and codeine to manage coughing is a decision that needs to be made by you and your doctor.

Other COPD drugs

Other medications are important for COPD management but don't affect the cough. These include:

corticosteroids, such as prednisone

long-acting anticholinergics, such as tiotropium (Spiriva), which can make the cough reflex more sensitive

Both prednisone and tiotropium can helpTrusted Source reduce cough due to COPD exacerbations.

Can you have COPD without a cough?

COPD includes both chronic bronchitis and emphysema.

Chronic bronchitis typically results in coughing and excess mucus production. Emphysema results in shortness of breath due to progressive destruction of alveoli, or air sacs, in the lungs. Shortness of breath rather than a cough is the most prominent symptom of emphysema. However, most patients with emphysema also have chronic bronchitis and therefore cough.

COPD and Diet: What to Eat and Avoid

It's always important to stick to a healthy and balanced diet, but especially so when you have underlying medical conditions. While you may not initially think food influences the symptoms of a lung condition like chronic obstructive pulmonary disease (COPD), it actually can. Your body uses food as fuel for all of its activities—breathing included. Therefore, eating the right foods and avoiding the wrong ones can ensure that you feel your best while coping with COPD.

What to Eat With COPD

Living with COPD can be difficult, but some strategies—like following a diet—can make it more comfortable. While a healthy diet won't cure COPD, it can help you feel your best by providing you with plenty of immune-boosting nutrients. So, what should you eat while dealing with COPD?

Protein

One of the main symptoms of COPD is fatigue. To help boost your energy, you should provide your body with ample amounts of protein. Plenty of foods are packed with protein, like milk, eggs, cheese, meat, fish, poultry, nuts, and dried beans.

Complex Carbohydrates

You should incorporate carbohydrates into your diet, but not simple ones—they are essentially sugar and do little for your body. Complex carbs, on the other hand, contain more nutrients and are therefore better for you. These can be found in foods like whole-wheat bread, quinoa, barley, potatoes, and sweet potatoes.

Potassium-Rich Foods

Potassium is a mineral that helps your muscles contract and nerves to function. Without enough potassium, your lungs may not expand and contract properly—a risk that those with COPD can't afford. You'll want to provide your body with plenty of potassium for proper lung function. Try to incorporate foods such as avocados, asparagus, beets, and dark leafy greens.

Foods to Avoid

With COPD, it's just as important to avoid certain foods. For an overall healthier lifestyle, you should steer clear of:

Salt

You should monitor salt or sodium intake, as it causes water retention which may affect your ability to breathe. While you put down the salt shaker, you should also check food labels to make sure they don't already have too much sodium.

Fried Foods

Any sort of food that is fried or greasy, like fast food, can cause bloating and discomfort, pushing on the diaphragm and making it harder to breathe.

Acidic Foods & Drinks

Consuming too many acidic foods and drinks can lead to heartburn and acid reflux. While this is uncomfortable on its own, acid reflux can also increase or worsen symptoms of COPD. So, it's best to limit acidic foods and drinks in your diet, like citrus, fruit juice, tomato sauce, coffee, and spicy foods.

Managing Your COPD Exacerbations

While you can follow these diet tips and take other measures to keep your symptoms of COPD under control, flare-ups can still occur. When these exacerbations do happen, you don't need to burden yourself with driving to the doctor—you can have DispatchHealth come to your home for prompt, professional care. We can assess your COPD exacerbations and help alleviate them through the necessary means, all while you're in the comfort of your own home.

Simple Carbohydrates vs. Complex Carbohydrates

Carbohydrates are a macronutrient found in a variety of food sources. There are several types, which can differ in terms of nutritional value and effects on health. Carbohydrates are a major macronutrient and one of your body's primary sources of energy. Some weight loss programs discourage eating them, but the key is finding the right carbs — not avoiding them completely. You may have heard that eating complex carbs is better than simple carbs. But nutrition labels don't always tell you if the carbohydrate content is simple or complex.

Complex carbohydrates are digested more slowly and release glucose into the blood stream more gradually. Simple carbohydrates are digested quickly and spike blood sugar faster and higher. Understanding how these foods are classified and how they work in your body can help you choose the right carbs.

Understanding carbohydrates

Carbohydrates are an important nutrient found in numerous types of foods. Most of us equate carbs with bread and pasta, but you can also find them in:

dairy products

fruits

vegetables

grains

nuts

legumes

seeds

sugary foods and sweets

Carbohydrates are made up of three components: fiber, starch, and sugar. Fiber and starch are complex carbs, while sugar is a simple carb. Depending on how much of each of these is found in a food determines its nutrient quality.

Simple carbs equal simplistic nutrition

Simple carbs are sugars. While some of these occur naturally in milk, most of the simple carbs in the American diet are added to foods. Common simple carbs added to foods include:

raw sugar

brown sugar

corn syrup and high-fructose corn syrup

glucose, fructose, and sucrose

fruit juice concentrate

Simple carb foods to limit

Try to avoid some of the most common refined sources of simple carbs and look for alternatives to satisfy those sweet cravings:

1. Soda

Sugary soda is bad for your health in several ways. You can try water flavored with lemon instead.

2. Baked treats

Satisfy your sweet tooth with fruit, rather than baked goods full of simple carbs and added sugars.

3. Packaged cookies

Bake your own goods using substitutes like applesauce or sweeteners, or look for other mixes that contain more complex carbs.

4. Fruit juice concentrate

An easy way to avoid fruit concentrate is to look closely at nutrition labels. Always choose 100 percent fruit juice or make your own at home.

5. Breakfast cereal

Breakfast cereals tend to be loaded with simple carbohydrates. If you just can't kick the habit, check out our rundown of breakfast cereals, from the best to the worst for your health.

THE MORE COMPLEX THE CARB, THE BETTER

Complex carbs pack in more nutrients than simple carbs. They're higher in fiber and digest more slowly. This also makes them more filling, which means they're a good option for weight control. They're also ideal for people with type 2 diabetes because they help manage blood sugar spikes after meals. Fiber and starch are the two types of complex carbohydrates. Fiber is especially important because it promotes bowel regularity and helps to control cholesterol. The main sources of dietary fiber include:

fruits

vegetables

nuts

beans

whole grains

Starch is also found in some of the same foods as fiber. The difference is certain foods are considered more starchy than fibrous, such as potatoes.

Other high-starch foods are:

whole wheat bread

cereal

corn

oats

peas

rice

Complex carbohydrates are key to long-term health. They make it easier to maintain a healthy weight and can even help guard against type 2 diabetes and cardiovascular problems in the future.

Complex carbs you should eat more of

Be sure to include the following complex carbohydrates as a regular part of your diet:

1. Whole grains

Whole grains are good sources of fiber, as well as potassium, magnesium, and selenium. Choose less processed whole grains such as quinoa, buckwheat, and whole-wheat pasta.

2. Fiber-rich fruits

Some of these are apples, berries, and bananas. Avoid canned fruit since it usually contains added syrup.

3. Fiber-rich vegetables

Eat more of all your veggies, including broccoli, leafy greens, and carrots.

4. Beans

Aside from fiber, these are good sources of folate, iron, and potassium. Choosing the right carbs can take time and practice. With a little bit of research and a keen eye for nutrition labels, you can start making healthier choices to energize your body and protect it from long-term complications.

WHAT'S IN A CARB?
Carbs are made up of fiber, starch, and sugars. The American Diabetes Association recommends getting 25 to 35 grams of fiber per day.

Recipes

Chicken pasta bake
Preparation and cooking time

Prep:30 mins

Cook:45 mins

Easy

Serves 6

Enjoy this gooey cheese and chicken pasta bake for the ultimate weekday family dinner. Serve straight from the dish with a dressed green salad

Nutrition: Per serving

NutrientUnit

kcal

575

fat

30g

saturates

14g

carbs

41g

sugars

9g

fibre

5g

protein

33g

salt

0.5g

Ingredients

4 tbsp olive oil

1 onion, finely chopped

2 garlic cloves, crushed

¼ tsp chilli flakes

2 x 400g cans chopped tomatoes

1 tsp caster sugar

6 tbsp mascarpone

4 skinless chicken breasts, sliced into strips

300g penne

70g mature cheddar, grated

50g grated mozzarella

½ small bunch of parsley, finely chopped

Method

STEP 1

Heat 2 tbsp of the oil in a pan over a medium heat and fry the onion gently for 10-12 mins. Add the garlic and chilli flakes and cook for 1 min. Tip in the tomatoes and sugar and season to taste. Simmer uncovered for 20 mins or until thickened, then stir through the mascarpone.

STEP 2

Heat 1 tbsp of oil in a non-stick frying pan. Season the chicken and fry for 5-7 mins or until the chicken is cooked through.

STEP 3

Heat the oven to 220C/200C fan/gas 7. Cook the penne following pack instructions. Drain and toss with the remaining oil. Tip the pasta into a medium sized ovenproof dish. Stir in the chicken and pour over the sauce. Top with the cheddar, mozzarella and parsley. Bake for 20 mins or until golden brown and bubbling.

Air-fryer soy & cranberry chicken wings
Preparation and cooking time

Prep:5 mins

Cook:20 mins - 40 mins

Easy

Serves 8

Marinate chicken wings in cranberry and soy sauce, then cook in an air-fryer to make this tasty side. They're perfect for a buffet or movie night snack

Nutrition: Per serving

NutrientUnit

kcal

187

fat

10g

saturates

3g

carbs

8g

sugars

7g

fibre

0.4g

protein

16g

salt

0.8g

Ingredients

1kg chicken wings

3 tbsp soy sauce

6 tbsp cranberry sauce

1 tsp dried oregano

2 garlic cloves, crushed

2 tsp ginger paste or freshly grated ginger

2 tsp vegetable oil

Method

STEP 1

Pat the chicken wings dry using a clean tea towel or kitchen paper (this helps ensure the wings crisp up). Heat the air-fryer to 200C. Combine the soy sauce, cranberry sauce, oregano, garlic, ginger and vegetable oil in a small bowl or jug. Put the chicken wings in a large bowl, then spoon or pour over the cranberry mixture.

STEP 2

Toss everything together and mix well so the chicken wings are well coated. The uncooked wings will keep frozen in an airtight container for up to three months. Tip the wings into the air-fryer basket and cook for 15-20 mins at 200C (or 20-25 mins at 180C from frozen), turning halfway through until cooked through and beginning to brown at the edges. You may need to do this in two batches depending on the size of your air-fryer.

Olive-brine chicken
Preparation and cooking time

Prep:20 mins

Cook:45 mins

plus at least 8 hrs brining

Easy

Serves 4

Beat food waste and use up olive brine to make this flavourful chicken dinner. Nocellara olives work well, but any green olives will do

Gluten-free

Nutrition: Per serving

NutrientUnit

kcal

613

fat

48g

saturates

16g

carbs

2g

sugars

1g

fibre

1g

protein

41g

salt

2g

Ingredients

1kg skin-on, bone-in chicken thighs

75g Nocellara olives, or any green olives, smashed, reserving 150ml brine from the jar

2 tbsp olive oil

4 garlic cloves, finely sliced

2 shallots, cut into rings

1 lemon, 1/2 juiced, 1/2 sliced

50g unsalted butter

small handful of parsley, finely chopped

new potatoes or rice, to serve

Method

STEP 1

Tip the chicken and olive brine into a freezer bag or baking dish, making sure the chicken is as submerged as possible. Cover and leave in the fridge overnight for at least 8 hrs or up to 12 hrs.

STEP 2

Heat the olive oil in a heavy-based saucepan over a medium-high heat. Remove the thighs from the brine, shaking off the excess and add to the pan, skin-side down. Fry for 10-15 mins until golden and crispy. You may need to do this in batches. Flip the thighs and sprinkle the smashed olives, garlic, shallots, lemon slices and butter into the pan along with a good splash of water. Continue to cook for a further 10-15 mins, until the chicken is cooked through. Pour in some water if it starts to look too dry. Add a splash of lemon juice and season to taste, adding more lemon juice if you prefer. Spoon the pan juices over the chicken to serve and scatter over the parsley. Serve with some crushed new potatoes or rice, if you like.

Grilled langoustines with citrus-dressed samphire, courgette and couscous salad
Preparation time

less than 30 mins

Cooking time

10 to 30 mins

Serves

Serves 2

A lovely fresh seafood dish for summer that, once you've got the blanching out the way, is pretty quick to put together.

Ingredients

6 langoustines

150g/5½oz samphire

1 courgette, thinly sliced

1 orange, zest and juice

1 lemon, zest and juice

4 tbsp olive oil

75g/2½oz couscous

1 tbsp harissa paste

3 tbsp pine nuts

2 tbsp chopped fresh coriander

Method

Bring a pan of boiling salted water to the boil, add the langoustines and blanch for about 20 seconds, then remove from the pan and transfer to a bowl of ice cold water. Remove the head and claws, and crack the shell to peel it away. De-vein by removing the black intestinal tract using a sharp knife. Set aside.

Heat a pan of boiling water in a medium pan and blanch the samphire for a couple of minutes. Remove and set aside.

Toss the thin sliced courgettes and cooled samphire in the citrus juice and 2 tablespoons of the olive oil in a bowl. Add salt, to taste, and leave to steep for 5 minutes.

In a bowl, pour boiling water over the couscous and the harissa paste. Cover and allow to absorb for 5–10 minutes. Stir in the remaining 2 tablespoons of olive oil, salt and the citrus zest.

Heat a pan over a medium heat and dry fry the pine nuts until nicely toasted. Set aside.

Heat a grill to hot, and then grill the langoustines for a few minutes on both sides.

To serve, scatter the courgettes and samphire on a plate, spoon

Weeping tiger fillet steak with noodles and shrimps
Preparation time

over 2 hours

Cooking time

10 to 30 mins

Serves

Serves 2

Fillet steak stands up to the powerful but perfectly balanced Thai flavours in this simple, impressive dish.

Ingredients

For the steak

3 tbsp Thai fish sauce

1 tbsp dark soy sauce

2 tsp dark brown soft sugar

2 garlic cloves, crushed

¼ tsp ground coriander

¼ tsp ground black pepper

2 x 175g/6oz fillet steaks

groundnut oil, for cooking

For the dressing

2 tbsp rice wine vinegar

1 tablespoon lime juice

2 tsp Thai fish sauce

2 tsp light brown soft sugar

1 tbsp chopped fresh coriander

1 tsp tamarind paste

1 red chilli, finely chopped

For the noodles

150g/5½oz dried egg noodles

2 tbsp sesame oil

1 tbsp groundnut oil

1 tbsp chopped red chilli

150g/5½oz cooked shrimps

1 tbsp chopped fresh coriander

2 spring onions, thinly sliced

1 tbsp light soy sauce

pinch sea salt

pinch ground ginger

Method

Mix all the steak ingredients except the meat and oil together in a bowl until the sugar has dissolved.

Place the steak in a sealable bag, add the marinade and gently massage it into the meat. Seal the bag with no air inside it and leave to marinate in the fridge for 6–8 hours.

To make the dressing, warm the vinegar, lime juice and fish sauce in a small saucepan over a low heat. Add the sugar and stir until dissolved, then stir in the coriander, tamarind paste and red chilli.

Half an hour before cooking, remove the steak from the bag and pat it dry with kitchen paper.

Place a griddle pan over a high heat and carefully rub it with groundnut oil using kitchen paper. Cook the steak for

2 minutes on each side, then turn it and cook for another minute, or until browned. Remove it from the pan and leave it to rest for 10 minutes.

Meanwhile, cook the noodles in a saucepan of boiling water for 2 minutes, then drain and set aside. Heat the sesame and groundnut oils in a large frying pan over a medium heat. Add the chilli and shrimps and cook for 3–4 minutes. Add the noodles, coriander and spring onions and stir in the soy sauce. Season with salt and ginger.

To serve, place a twist of noodles on the plate. Slice the steak thinly and place it next to the noodles. Spoon some of the dressing over the noodles and serve

Caribbean rice and beans
Preparation time

less than 30 mins

Cooking time

30 mins to 1 hour

Serves

Serves 6

Dietary

Vegetarian

This recipe uses the most popular beans in a Caribbean kitchen (black beans and kidney beans), all cooked up in a turmeric paste which adds extra flavour to the soft fluffy rice.

Each serving provides 533 kcal, 15g protein, 84g carbohydrates (of which 7g sugars), 12.5g fat (of which 7g saturates), 11g fibre and 1.3g salt.

Ingredients

2 tbsp vegetable oil

1 large brown onion, chopped

3 spring onions, finely chopped

4 garlic cloves, finely chopped

thumb-sized piece fresh root ginger, peeled and finely chopped

½ Scotch bonnet chilli, seeds removed, finely chopped

2 tbsp ground turmeric

1 carrot, finely chopped

400g tin chopped tomatoes

200g tin coconut milk

400g tin black beans, drained and rinsed

400g tin kidney beans, drained and rinsed

1½ tsp sea salt flakes

1 tsp freshly ground black pepper

500g/1lb 2oz white or brown rice, rinsed

5 fresh thyme sprigs

1 tbsp butter

fresh flatleaf parsley, finely chopped, to garnish

squeeze lemon juice, to serve

Method

Heat the oil in a large frying pan over a low heat. Add the onion, spring onions, garlic, ginger, Scotch bonnet and turmeric. Fry for 3 minutes, until the onion and garlic are softened.

Add the carrot, tomatoes, coconut milk, black beans, kidney beans, salt and pepper and bring to the boil. Add the rice, mix and, if necessary, add more water so the liquid level is just above the rice. Add the thyme and butter and bring to the boil. Reduce the heat to low, cover with a lid and simmer for 25 minutes, or until the water is fully absorbed and the rice cooked through.

Garnish with the parsley, add the squeeze of lemon juice and serve.

Beanie burgers
Preparation time

less than 30 mins

Cooking time

less than 10 mins

Serves

Serves 4

Dietary

Vegetarian

Turn a tin of kidney beans into a gently spicy and budget-friendly veggie burger that you can whip up in 20 minutes.

Ingredients

For the burgers

1 large potato (about 285g/10oz), peeled and cut into large chunks

400g tin red kidney beans, drained and rinsed

1 small red onion, finely chopped

1 tsp salt

½ tsp dried chilli flakes

1 tsp ground cumin

1 slice bread (about 65g/2¼oz), blitzed to crumbs (see recipe tip)

3–4 tbsp vegetable oil

To serve

4 burger buns, cut in half

3–4 ripe tomatoes, sliced

shredded iceberg lettuce

sauces of your choice, such as mayonnaise, mustard or ketchup (optional)

Recipe tips

Method

Place the potato in a pan of boiling water and simmer for 12–15 minutes, or until very tender but not breaking apart. Drain well and leave to air dry for a few minutes.

In a bowl, mash the rinsed beans using a potato masher. Add the potatoes and mash those too. Mix in the remaining burger ingredients, except the oil. Shape the mixture into four large patties.

Heat 2 tablespoons of oil in a large frying pan (preferably non-stick). Cook the burgers over a medium heat for 3–4 minutes on each side until golden, adding a little extra oil when the burgers are turned.

Toast the buns, in a dry frying pan or griddle, cut-side down and divide between four plates. Add lettuce and tomatoes, if using. Top with the hot burgers and serve with sauces of your choice.

Recipe Tips

If you have any leftover mashed potato feel free to use that instead of boiling and mashing another potato.

To make fresh breadcrumbs without a food processor, freeze the bread until solid and then grate.

You can use the same frying pan to toast the buns as you use to cook the burgers as they don't take long. I

Blackened beef with pickled red cabbage and miso herb butter
Preparation time

over 2 hours

Cooking time

1 to 2 hours

Serves

Serves 2

Smoky blackened beef, the tang of pickled cabbage and a rich miso butter spooned over the top – this recipe has it all!

Ingredients

For the beef rump cap

1 beef rump cap, around 1kg/2lb 4oz in weight

2 tbsp olive oil

For the spice rub

4 tbsp salt

4 tbsp hot smoked paprika

3 tbsp soft brown sugar

2 tbsp coarse ground black pepper

2 tbsp garlic powder

2 tbsp onion powder

2 tbsp dried oregano

2 tbsp dried thyme

2 tbsp cep or mushroom powder

2 tbsp powdered cumin

For the pickled red cabbage

2 tsp salt

½ red cabbage, shredded

1 tbsp coriander seeds

3 tbsp cashew nuts

2 lemongrass sticks, smashed

250ml/9fl oz red wine vinegar

100g/3½oz caster sugar

2 Cox apples, julienned

1 tsp roasted sesame seeds

For the miso herb butter

100g/3½oz unsalted butter

75g/2½oz white miso paste

2 tbsp coriander, chopped

1 green chilli, finely diced

1 lime, juice and zest

1 garlic clove, minced

Method

Rub the oil into the beef cap. Mix the dry spices together, and rub the spice mix generously into the meat. Leave to marinate for a few hours.

Combine the salt and the shredded cabbage and transfer to a colander. Leave for an hour to allow some of the excess moisture to drain out of the cabbage.

Toast the coriander seeds and cashew nuts in a hot pan or in the oven. Crush the coriander seeds and roughly chop the cashew nuts.

Combine the coriander seeds, lemongrass, vinegar and sugar together in a pan and bring to the boil. Once the sugar has dissolved, drop the cabbage into the pickling liquor and remove from the heat. Allow the cabbage to cool in the liquor then drain and toss with the apple, cashews and sesame seeds.

Preheat the oven to 200C/180C Fan/Gas 6

Heat a frying pan over a medium-high heat, and sear the rump cap all over to give it a nice crust and colour. Transfer the rump cap to the oven for 15–20 minutes, depending on the thickness.

For the herb butter, mix all the ingredients together and set aside.

To serve, slice the beef and spoon over some of the softened herb butter. Pile the red cabbage on the side.

Braised feather blade beef
Preparation time: 30 mins to 1 hour

Cooking time:over 2 hours

Serves: Serves 2–4

Here, beef is slow cooked in a savoury, spicy sauce in the oven before being served with chargrilled, marinated carrots and parsnips.

Ingredients

For the beef

2 tbsp olive oil

1kg/2lb 4oz feather blade beef

2 onions, sliced

2 garlic bulbs, cut in half

1 tbsp coriander seeds

1 tsp cumin seeds

1 tsp Chinese five-spice powder

2 star anise

1 litre/1¾ pint beef stock

1 tbsp soy sauce

2 tbsp honey

salt and freshly ground black pepper

For the carrots and parsnips

3 young heritage carrots, peeled and left whole

3 young parsnips, peeled and left whole

4 tbsp soy sauce

4 tbsp rice wine vinegar

2 garlic cloves, minced

3 tbsp sesame oil

1 tbsp minced fresh root ginger

¼ tsp Chinese five-spice powder

salt

1 tbsp snipped fresh chives, to serve

Method

To make the beef, preheat the oven to 180C/160C Fan/Gas 4. Heat the oil in a casserole, season the beef well and cook in the pan until coloured all over. Remove from the pan.

Sweat the onion, garlic bulbs and spices in the casserole for 10 minutes. Add the stock, soy sauce and honey and add the beef back in. Cook in the oven for around 3½ hours until the beef is tender.

To make the carrots and parsnips, cook them in a saucepan of boiling salted water until just tender. Combine the soy sauce, vinegar, garlic, sesame oil, ginger and five-spice powder in a large bowl and add the cooked carrots and parsnips. Mix and leave to marinate for 30 minutes.

Heat a griddle pan on high heat, and char the vegetables for 2 minutes all over.

To serve, toss the carrots and parsnips in the chives and serve with the beef and some of the cooking liquor.

9 798872 634393